MARK WILLIAM KANTER
&
PINK PUPPY PUBLISHING
Presents

THE
10 DAY
COLITIS CURE

HOW I
CURED 10 YEARS OF COLITIS
BY CHRISTMAS

I0425067

For Ulcerative Colitis sufferers everywhere.
I believe you can cure yourself like I did.

CHAPTERS

Chapter 1

Whadya Mean – I've got Ulcerative Colitis?

When I was about 30 years old, I moved from New Jersey to Arizona in search of better weather, a better career and as an escape from a failed business venture. I left my friends and parents behind and entered the computer programming profession, of which, I knew very little at the time.

The stress was significant, yet I kept it inside. At my new day job, I started binging on coffee with lots of milk and sugar, probably 5 – 10 cups a day. It was my vice to get through the day. I studied like mad on my off time to learn the ins and outs of programming.

My new job was a big switch for me, both mentally and physically. I had gone from Mr Outdoors, Mr Independent, to Mr Stuck-in-a-Cube, Mr Work-for-the-Man. I struggled daily with the thought of, "Is this it? This is what I do for the rest of my life?"

I also loaded up on pizza, 4-5 slices at a time and a six pack of beer on the weekends. At that time, I weighed about 170 pounds, which was about normal for my height of 5 foot 7 inches.

The stress of this change, a sedentary lifestyle, and a poor diet, quickly took a toll on me and when the flu went around the office, I caught it, but good! I went on a dose or 2 of antibiotics, and finally got through the cold that had kept me out of work for a couple of weeks.

During that first summer in Arizona, the weather swelled to over 120 degrees and lasted that way for an entire week. At that point, I knew Arizona was not going to work out for me and I started making plans to move to San Diego, CA, where the weather was supposedly much better, but the cost of living was much higher.

Two weeks before the move to San Diego, something pretty alarming happened to me. I went to the bathroom and after my bowel movement, I looked in the bowl and saw bright red blood - about a teaspoons worth.

I still knew only a little about programming and worried about how I was going to get a job and afford living in San Diego. On top of that, I now had to deal with blood in my stool.

Nevertheless, I moved to San Diego and landed a job with a startup company as a consultant and began working 100 hour weeks. Again I was binging on coffee, with lots of milk and sugar, while I tried to learn as much as I could on my off time to catch up on the programming skills I felt I lacked.

Over the next few months , the bleeding progressed. Eventually, at every movement, there was blood in the bowl - about 1-2 tablespoons worth.

I tried adding a salad to my otherwise crappy daily diet. That seemed to help for a short while, but I kept working crazy hours and binged on coffee, pizza and beer, more and more.

PAIN KICKS IN

And then, the pain and urgency kicked in. Suddenly I found myself running to the bathroom, having to leave meetings suddenly. Several times I didn't make it in time and soiled my pants. Yet, somehow I was able to keep this embarrassing truth away from the eyes of my associates.

The stress mounted as now I had to contend with keeping an eye out for the nearest bathroom wherever I went . I was afraid to go for a ride in anybodies car as I might have to go to the bathroom suddenly and not be able to get out of the car. At this point, I was going to the bathroom about 5-10 times a day. It smelled really foul and hurt more and more. I also began seeing white mucous mixed in with the blood.

Every time I ate, my stomach grumbled loud enough for my associates to hear. Within minutes of eating, I had to run, sometimes after the very first bite.

DOCTOR SHOCK

I finally made the time to go get it checked out by a doctor. It was my wifes birthday. I went to an emergency room and the attending took a look in my rectum with a long snakelike tube of some sort. I think he was an intern, because he started to panic. I remember him having blood on his gloves and suddenly talking really loud during the exam. "We've got blood here, a lot of blood! Somebody page Dr. Baldy!" I call him

Baldy, because I don't remember the Doctors name, I just remember he was Bald. And he was kinda cold. Reminded me of this childhood memory where a neighborhood kid used to call this guy down the street "Baldy" and the guy would chase the kid. That guy was cold too.

Anyhow, Dr Baldy arrived about 10 minutes later, all the while I am lying on my side, 3 nurses in the room, with an intern holding this snake in my butt, panicking. What fun that was, let me tell you. On top of it, the guy kept pumping air inside me, to allow the snake to move easier, but it was causing me extreme pain, I felt like I was gonna blast him and the entire room with feces! But I had to hold it. It pains me just thinking about that day.

Dr Baldy checked things out,. He did a biopsy and told me I have Ulcerative Colitis. The intern wrote me a prescription for Asacol and gave me a brief description of what Ulcerative Colitis was. He said, it just means I have to take these pills every day to keep it under control and get a colonoscopy checkup every year. He spoke as if it was no big deal.

I wanted to believe that, but more so, I felt really alone, and didn't feel like I was being given any emotional support by the system. I had lots of questions, but it was clear to me they did not want to spend the time answering them and I was sent on my way. I was interfering with their other patients. They were done with me. It was all so cold feeling.

On top of that, I was still very concerned with learning the programming skills I needed so I could keep my job and continue to afford living in San Diego. But now I had to go research what the heck Ulcerative Colitis was and what could be done about it, as I did not want to blindly follow one doctors opinion. The stress amplified.

I remember agonizing about going home to tell my wife, "Happy Birthday Honey, I have Ulcerative Colitis."

My wife loves roller coaster rides. But little did we know then, that we just boarded one of the worlds most challenging roller coasters ever - one that would keep us dizzy for the next 10 years of our lives and seriously strain our marriage

So, off to a library we went, reading up on this thing called Ulcerative Colitis. And what we learned was not very encouraging. Here's what all the texts basically said,

"Ulcerative Colitis, also considered an Inflammatory Bowel Disease or IBD, is a chronic auto immune condition affecting the large intestines, whereby the body mistakenly attacks the inner walls of the large intestine, causing painful inflammation, mucous and ulcerations of the intestine, leading to bloody, mucous-laden and foul-smelling stools, urgent and frequent bowel movements, 5-10 times a day or more, and a decreased ability to absorb nutrients from food, resulting in significant weight loss over time and an increased risk of colon cancer after 10 years.

Approximately 500,000 people in the United States are currently living with Ulcerative Colitis. About 30,000 new cases are diagnosed each year The cause of Ulcerative Colitis is unknown."

Chapter 2

Whadya Mean – Cause Unknown?

So, the body supposedly just wakes up one day and decides to attack itself for no reason at all? C'mon! I don't buy it.

Yet, everything I read said the same thing, that this was an autoimmune disorder. But I kept thinking... that's a cop out. These books are written by a world that just does not know yet what causes Colitis.

I am a firm believer that everything happens for a reason - for every effect, there is a cause.

ELEMENTARY MY DEAR WATSON

For example. if a plate shatters on the floor, its because somebody dropped the plate. If somebody dropped a plate, it's because their hands were slippery. If somebodies hands were slippery, it's because they just washed them and didn't dry them. If they didn't dry them, it's because they were in a hurry. If they were in a hurry, its because they left late. If they left late, it's because they slept through their alarm clock. If they slept through their alarm clock, it's because they stayed up late watching Conan O'brien or some other show - etc, etc. You get the idea. So when the plate broke, one could reasonably deduce – "If he only would have went to bed on time last night, none of this would have happened."

So, nothing happens without something first causing it to happen. To hear that the body just attacks itself for no known reason... that's just rubbish to me! And it gave me great hope that a cause just needed to be discovered. But it also left me disheartened as I felt the industry had given up trying to find the cause. It was as if the guy who broke the plate said, "Those darn plates, I hate it when they do that!"

A BITTERSWEET TRUTH

Why would anyone in the medical industry try to find and prevent people from getting Colitis? After all, Colitis is great for business. People don't usually die from it and they will buy medicine every month that tries to keep it under control for 10 years or more, plus they will keep coming back for a Colonoscopy each year. And at some point, 40 percent of them will opt to have surgery to remove the large intestine that finally becomes completely affected and useless or develops cancer Why would anyone in the medical industry want to turn off that revenue stream?

If I was in that industry, I wouldn't want to turn off that revenue stream . And actually, I am quite thankful that the pharmaceutical companies provided the drug Asacol, which gave me some relief along the way.

I can't imagine how I would have survived without it early on.

I am also thankful that early on, when I was pretty much in shock, doctors gave me steroids to give me a boost.

Further, when my iron count fell dangerously low, due to the constant bleeding, it was the doctors at the emergency rooms who brought me back from near death with their infusions, injections and bedside sympathy.

ON A PORCELAIN HORSE I RIDE

Being from New Jersey, obviously I am a big fan of Jon Bon Jovi and funny enough, like his song <u>Wanted Dead or Alive,</u> I found myself a cowboy but instead of riding a steel horse, I was riding on toilet bowls wherever I went. All the while, I was trying to find a cause and cure for this without much help from the industry.

After the fact,. some of the stuff that happened along the way, can be looked back on and laughed at.

I remember thinking, "I should write a book about public restrooms. A guide to the best and worst," because I'd seen them all. I've been to ones in every restaurant, in every hospital, in every gas station, in every office building, in every amusement park, in every casino, everywhere, at least 5 times a year.

I am a public restroom expert. Maybe I could be a restroom designer? Oh and the stories I could tell about the sounds I've heard in them, or the sounds I've made in them.

Oh and then there were the times I couldn't find a restroom in time. You've heard the phrase: "Does a Bear Sh*t in the woods?" well I have my own embarrassing version: "Does an Ulcerative Colitis Patient Sh*t in the middle of a Crowded Street?" As Sarah Palin might say: "You betcha!"

I AM RESPONSIBLE

So digression aside, and despite my feeling alone in the quest for a cause, I am ever the optimist and I felt, I did this to myself. Somehow, I can undo this.

I went to Naturalopaths, Gastroenterologists, and Acupuncturists, but no one had the answers to what caused Colitis or at least, no answer I could believe at the time.

They ran tests after tests. Everything was consistent with a diagnosis of Ulcerative Colitis. They said it wasn't an infection, it wasn't an allergy, it wasn't a virus, it wasn't anything but Ulcerative Colitis.

One test however, by Dr Mark Stengler and Great Smokies Lab, turned out to be very key to my finding my cure, but I will get to that later.

(Thank you Dr Stengler & Great Smokies)

Several years slipped by and I was not having luck in finding the cause of the illness and so I changed my focus onto finding a cure, which, looking back now, was a fruitless endeavor. How can you cure something without knowing the underlying cause? If you don't know the underlying cause, how can you ever cure it? And the answer is, you can't. At least I couldn't.

It wasn't until 10 years later that I would focus with extreme intensity on the cause of the disease, that I would finally figure it out.

But anyway, with my focus changed to cures., I read with intensity. Unfortunately, everything I read said that there is no known cure for colitis.

The best I could find was statements saying that when the Large Intestine is removed surgically, the patient no longer suffers from Colitis.

THE ABC's OF SURGERY
Today's letter is J

When I looked into what the surgery entailed in my 111th year of the disease, turns out, it is something I would only opt for as a last resort only if I couldn't survive or cope without removing it. And according to a visit with my Colorectal Surgeon, this is typically the case in 40% of Ulcerative Colitis at some point or another.

The surgeon told me if I elect to have surgery he would recommend J Pouch Surgery. It entails removing the large intestine entirely. Then he would take the end of the small intestine and bend it up toward itself forming a letter J.

He would stitch the J shape in place to itself, and then cut open the bottom of the J. This forms a pouch that will serve as a small reservoir, similar to what the rectum does. He would then stitch the opening of the J Pouch to the little bit of Rectum he left behind when he removed the Large intestine.

This takes place at 2 different surgeries. The first one removes the intestine and stitches the J Pouch to a small hole in the stomach that then goes to a plastic bag the patient has to carry on his outside. The bag collects poop and the patient has to clean it out regularly. (JOY)

The bag stays like that for 2-3 months allowing time for the J pouch stitches to heal. Once they are healed, then the second surgery closes the hole in the stomach and moves the J Pouch down and connects it to the leftover Rectum.

"SERIOUSLY?"

The entire cast of Grey's Anatomy

So, with every surgery, there are risks, complications, and expectations. Here's what I was told could happen and what I could expect, that is, after I got passed the grossness of imagining living with a bag of poop under my shirt for 3 months. (Who wants to give Daddy a great big hug? Anybody? Anybody?)

I could expect that first, I would be in the hospital for 1 week for the first surgery. I will be out of work for about a month as I will be very tired all the time. I will need to pump myself up with pain medication for the first week for certain.

I will be fed intravenously until my small intestines show signs of waking up. Apparently they go to sleep during the surgery and take a while to wake up, whatever that means.

I will have many tubes in me when I wake from surgery. One tube a day will be removed.

When I wake, I will have a bag attached to a hole in my stomach.

In 3 months I come back and spend 3 days in the hospital for the 2nd part of the procedure. I will be out of work for 2 weeks.

From here on out, I will likely go to the bathroom 4-8 times a day. It could be 12-15 times a day or more or it could be 2-3 times a day, but typically it's 4-8. The stools will never be formed, they will always be liquid, since the large intestine is what use to cause formed stool by allowing the water from the stool to be absorbed by the body through its walls. Without a large intestine, that can no longer happen and the bile and small-intestine-liquified food is all that I will see.

LEAKAGE? – WTF!

There is a chance of leakage, where I would have to go back in for surgery to repair things. This is when the stitches don't heal fully and poop goes right into the bloodstream. (JOY)

There is a regular chance of Pouchitis, which is a painful infection in the J Pouch area, that I will need to load up on antibiotics to help overcome. I will need to be careful what and how I eat so as not to make Pouchitis more likely.

There is a 25% chance that, due to nerves being severed during the procedure that removes most of the rectum and large intestine, that I will have trouble urinating and it will be painful. I will need to take medication everyday to help me urinate.

There is a 25% chance that I will have sexual dysfunction.

The most common side effects are Low Blood Counts and Kidney Complications.

Doesn't sound any better than what I had before surgery and it actually sounds much worse.

So in essence, according to the texts, there is no known cure. The closest, is cutting it out, only to trade the current problems for a different set of similar and possibly worse problems. The only upside is that with surgery, I might not have to get a colonoscopy anymore because without an intestine, you don't get colon cancer.

Chapter 3

Whadya Mean – No Known Cure?

"Whose in charge here? I demand to see the person in charge - somebody! How can there be no known cure for this? What have you people been doing for the last 50 years in the research department? I want somebody's butt! You're all FIRED!"

As if that's gonna get me anywhere. Well ,as one of my doctors recently wrote about me, "Patient needs to come to terms with this disease," Well, I have. And here are this patients terms.

I have come to terms with the fact that no one is coming to my aid to find or declare a definitive cause of Ulcerative Colitis and the only work being done in the field is to find drugs that help mask the symptoms and suppress the immune system. (And I can't blame them though.)

I've come to terms that if I want a cure, I need to fix the root cause.

I've come to terms that there are a bunch of drugs to help control symptoms, but I don't want to take drugs anymore and it hasn't been doing that well for me the past few years in particular. I don't want to ride the roller coaster anymore.

I've come to terms that I do not want to get a colonsocpy every year any more to check for cancer. Oh! Did I forget to mention the joys of a Colonoscopy? Every year, I had to have the snake inserted in my rectum and let them take pictures all the way through the large intestines.

YOU DIDN'T WANT THAT DID YOU?

During the Colonscopy, they also take biopsies, which is a nice way of saying, they pluck a nice chuck of my intestine off in several spots using an Alien tooth like device that shoots out of the snakes head and bites off a piece of my inner intestine wall and then goes back inside its nasty head. I actually was awake for one of these bites and felt it pull the chunk. I also saw the blood coming from the bite area afterwards. I'm sure *that* was good for me, NOT!

Actually, the doctors mean well, trying to screen for cancer early enough, however I often have more blood in the bowl for the next few days after the procedure.

And did I mention the best part. I get to drink poison the day before the procedure and starve myself until the procedure is done. The poison is this gallon of liquid stuff that I have to drink completely in 1 hour and it makes me have eruption-like diarrhea for the next 3 hours. It makes me want to die! No kidding.

I've come to terms that I do not want to get surgery to remove my intestine.

I've come to terms that I will find a definitive cause and a cure or I will die trying. (Fortunately, I found it, so now I can get busy living again.)

Early on I was told countless times, that, "Diet doesn't matter when it comes to Colitis. It doesn't really matter what you eat. You would have gotten this anyway and you will flair no matter what. It simply cycles, with periods of no or little symptoms to periods of severe symptoms. "

Recently I've been told "you might want to watch what you eat as certain things can make symptoms worse - it all depends on the person, everyone is different. Diet may or may not help."

How can diet not cause this, yet it can make symptoms worse? That doesn't add up to me.

I've come to terms that diet must have a causative role in this and that when I find out exactly how, I will have a basis to find a cure.

Chapter 4

Whadya Mean – Diet Doesn't Matter?

Talk about depression. Can you imagine being told it doesn't matter what you do, what you say, what you eat, you are going to get a terrible disease by the time you are 30, no matter what. You are genetically prone to it, case closed.

That's basically what I was told. It didn't matter what I did, some people just get it and others don't. I was the lucky 1 in 10,000 that get it every year.

Well I didn't want to believe that and if fact I certainly don't now, but at times, when that's what all the experts are telling you, you start to believe it and you start to give up hope.

Fortunately, my father instilled in me a "Don't Quit" attitude. He gave me a plaque when I was a little boy that had a poem with that title on it. He would read it to me and recite it from memory sometimes when we were out together. I loved that poem and would read it over and over. And I always wanted to make him proud.

My hope would wain periodically, but then I would get back on my feet and try again. It was a never ending roller coaster and unfortunately it drove my wife crazy.

I was constantly trying a new diet, a new vitamin plan, a new enzyme plan, a new homeopathic remedy. And I would go full force.

I'd stock up on stuff from the stores and try something for a week or 2 and make progress, only to be disappointed shortly after when symptoms would kick in again and I would go backwards . Unfortunately, each time I fell, I fell further and it got harder and harder to get back up.

My weight dropped to 135 pounds by year 10 and I was but a shadow of the man I used to be. A frail looking person, once a champion wrestler in high school, who bragged about how much they could lift and how they set the school record for chin ups.

That was no more. I was pretty weak now and my confidence was shot.

But my Dad's poem somehow kept me going.

DONT QUIT

"When things go wrong as they sometimes will
When the road your trudging seem all uphill
When care is pressing down a bit
Rest if you must, but don't you quit.

Life is erratic with its twists and its turns
As everyone of us sometimes learns
And many a failure turns about
When he might have won had he stuck it out

So stick to the fight when you're hardest hit
It's when things seem worst that you mustn't
quit
Cause often the goal is nearer than
It seems to a faint and faltering man
And sooner or later the one who wins
Is the one who thinks he can"

(Thank you Dad)

This experimenting went on for 10 years. I don't know exactly how much money I blew on that stuff. But I'm sure my wife could give you the list of things she's thrown out after I abandoned each experiment.

This seriously strained our marriage as my wife is of the frugal sort and likes to walk before she runs. I'm just the opposite. I go gull force, spend whatever, don't worry about it, and adjust course as necessary. It made for some interesting arguments to say the least.

The most frustrating part for her was that she never knew what to cook. I would sometimes announce out of nowhere to her, "No I'm not eating that anymore" and then a week later she'd see me eating that item. God bless her. I don't know how she put up with it all and stuck by my side, but she did.

(Thank you Karin)

So after all the experimenting I did with diet and such to try and combat the symptoms, glimmering patterns of hope began to emerge.

I really began to take serious notice of how everything I ate affected me

I knew that certain foods, if eaten too many times in a row, would cause symptoms, whereas if eaten only once a week, would not cause symptoms.

I knew that anytime I ate, shortly after, I would get the urge to go to the bathroom.

I knew that certain foods just did not sit well no matter what.

I knew that sometimes a certain combination at a meal would affect me, and other times it would not.

I knew that overeating would cause symptoms.

I knew that not eating at all for a day would result in no symptoms.

I BEG TO DIFFER

So in my mind, Diet definitely had some effect on my symptoms and some cause in this whole thing. There was some answer lurking in emerging patterns , I just didn't know how to look and didn't have the right focus at the time.

In around year 6 of this disease, I had listened to Tony Robbins tape series called Personal Power. And in his lessons he said that the mind will always give you an answer. The trick is to ask it the right questions.

It wasn't until year 11, faced with impending surgery, that I put it all together and started asking the right questions.

(Thank you Tony)

Chapter 5

What the Heck Can I Eat?

Tony taught me to teach my brain to assume there is always an answer to any question I ask. He said I should begin by asking a specific question and ending it with … "And have fun in the process?"

For example, "How can I cure myself of colitis *AND* have fun in the process?"

This supposedly sets the mind up for coming up with the actual answer or providing steps to take to get to the answer.

I started asking that question about my diet and began making progress.

Then I started asking myself, "How can I find out what causes Colitis *AND* have fun in the process?"

Well it turns out I have fun doing research and the answer my brain gave me, sent me back to the text books and back to test results from 10 years earlier and back to the internet where I started digging through scholarly articles. I dug and I dug and I read and I read, and I followed every possible cause for every possible symptom I was having and every complication that can arise from my disease, and finally, it happened. One day I followed a complication of Ulcerative Colitis called Oral Thrush and although I had dismissed it early on as not relevant or not plausible, I dug some more into Thrush.

But before I get further into that and the actual cure, let me tell you all the diets I have tried and later it will become clear why they did not work for me.

One of the first questions I had when I was diagnosed with this more than 10 years ago, was what can I eat? And I got different answers from everybody and none of the suggestions worked for me, though apparently they had worked for others.

I have tried Elaine Gotschall's, Specific Carbohydrate Diet or SCD.
This diet basically eliminated most carbohydrates from the diet and allowed all kinds of fats, and proteins, and certain carbohydrates

I have tried Eating as a Vegan

This diet allowed any fruits, vegetables, nuts and seeds, but no animal products.

I have tried the Atkins Diet Revolution
This is similar to SCD except the carbohydrates could be any kind so long as they were a very small portion of the diet

I have tried an All Fat, no Carb, no Protein diet. This was one that some people who can not digest protein, must stay on. It was mainly Hotdogs, Celery and Cream Cheese.

I have tried an All Raw Food Diet
On this you could eat any food you want so long as it has not been heated or processed in any way.

I have tried and All Organic Diet
On this you could eat anything you want so long as it did not contain pesticides or hormones.

I have tried pouring enzymes all over my food before eating.

I have tried following food combining principles.
With this you could eat anything so long as you don't mix certain foods with others at any one

meal. Example: Don't eat fruit at the same time as Meat.

I have tried eliminating all Night Shades
This meant I could eat anything but Eggplant, Tomatoes, Mushrooms, and Potatoes , Peppers, and Cherries

I have tried total elimination of all foods and one at a time re-introduction

I have tried eating foods cooked only microwave or only by broiling, or only by grilling, or only by boiling, or only by crock pot.

I have tried making my own dehydrated foods and eating only those.

STICK IT

By far, the hardest part of all the strategies was sticking to any one of them over a long period. I would seem to do well on some, but could not maintain it for very long. I would eventually crack for desire of some of the foods I was depriving myself of. And then I would binge on the forbidden foods.

I am convinced now, that it wasn't a matter of will power, it was a matter of survival. With each one of these diets, either I was not improving or I was not getting enough nutrients and my mind forced me to eventually go and get what I needed so my body could survive.

But at the time of each diet, I had a different opinion and it was a confidence killer. I had believed that it was a lack of willpower and I was just too weak to stick with it.

Another major problem with any thing I tried was that symptoms don't necessarily show up right away. It can take 12 hours or more for some food to make it to my large intestines and by then I forgot what I ate or did not eat that either helped or did not help – that either caused symptoms or did not.

I tried logging things down in a journal like all the texts suggest, but I just found it too hard to keep up with and too frustrating, having done it for almost 10 years without a clear solution. Plus, I had a job and family and a whole other life to attend to. I was always losing my notes or just not confident that keeping them was going to help get me the answers.

If I were ever asked to stick with a Diet again that was making me crazy with desire for other foods. I would politely tell that person to STICK IT!

If I am craving, then I am not getting what I need and the diet is not right – that's my opinion anyhow. 10 years of sticking to Diets that drove me crazy will do that to a person I guess. I've earned the right to say STICK IT.

SO STICK IT. There, I said it Thrice. I feel better now.

STICK IT – say it with me!

I now have a diet where I am not craving anything and I am healed, happy and growing stronger every day. The diet must be right or STICK IT!

I'll get to the diet a little later, but just so you know what I didn't know upfront., guess what happens after you have had Colitis for 10 years?

You get to find out what happens after 10 years.

It seemed no one out there or in the texts wants to reveal what happens after 10 years. I find it all too suspicious, but understandable

Chapter 6

What Happens After 10 Years?

Well, for me, it meant you end up weighing a lot less than you did at the beginning. You end up having little if any confidence. You wind up having blood in your stool all the time. You wind up becoming anemic. You wind up becoming dangerously low on iron. You wind up highly susceptible to colds and get sick for long periods of time. You end up going on a dose of antibiotics to kill the cold you catch, but subsequently you end up having the worst flare up of your life, so painful you wish you were dead. Forget about trying to sleep through the night. That doesn't happen. Oh but sleep is overrated, I forgot.

And then they tell you your surgical options, which have their own set of problems, or they tell you of new drug options that may be risky and have serious side effects, possibly causing cancer and certainly taxing your liver and further suppressing your immune system, so you can catch more colds easier and go on more antibiotics and then, due to the horrible flair ups they produce, you get to contemplate death over living, more and more..

Sorry, do I sound Bitter? Yeah, I'm letting it out a bit. Sorry. But Bitter, it turns out ironically, is part of the CURE.

BITTER (FOR LACK OF A BETTER WORD) IS GOOD

I have gone through the stages of depression at least a dozen times during my battle against Colitis. And like the Terminator said. "Anger is the most useful emotion."

It's when I get angry that I get up the courage to get back on my feet and try again. After 10 years, you can imagine the anger built up inside.

Conversations with God, questioning the purpose of life, fighting with loved ones and most importantly, severe pain. It all pushes you to an edge where you find yourself trying yet again, despite wishing you were dead.

In this case, it was the last push I needed to win. If I didn't win this time, that was it for me. I can't imagine I could have gotten off the canvas one more time. I would have stayed down for the count and I pray no one else ever has to reach that point. That's the main reason I am writing this book. I remember some study about suicide related to Ulcerative Colitis, and now I UNDERSTAND why. Pain is an incredible motivator.

Bitter as I am, it turns out there is a pattern to the foods that worked well. And those that do are the Bitter tasting ones! The lord works in mysterious ways.

(Thank you God)

Chapter 7

Whadya Mean – My Only Option is a Cancer Causing Drug or Surgery to Remove My Intestines, Causing More Problems?

"Dem's Fightin' Words!
Put em up. I'm gonna kick your ass."

So 10 years go by, I'm doing my best to stay alive and hoping all along that if I don't cure this, then at least when I make it to 10 years, I can have the intestine removed and live a somewhat normal life again.

But then I learn the news that that ain't the case.

You want to talk about anger! And on top of it, my Gastroenterologist is giving me grief about not sticking to the protocol of going to get blood work done regularly and missing appointments for the lovely Colonoscopy party. And if I would just try this one other new drug, it might help get it under control. What a bad patient I am.

Just what I needed to hear to get me fired up to fight back, and this time, finally win.

I'm sure he meant well and was practicing what he was taught, but if you listen to Dr Weil, you will learn that Doctors are not taught about preventive medicine, and the medical industry is basically not very good at fixing the underlying cause of so-called chronic auto-immune disorders, like arthritis, fibromyalgia, and colitis. They are great at acute problems, like surgery to reattach a limb or cut out diseased parts, or repair a heart. But long-term, systemic problems are a mystery in their world and my case is a perfect example.

FIGHT BACK

So I have my own option, different than what they proposed – and that is... Fight back! Cure this damn thing and write a book about it and put an end to the misery half a million people are suffering from and save the 30,000 more that get shocked into this roller coaster ride each year.

Chapter 8

Why Is God Giving Me All This Unbearable Pain – Why Doesn't He Just Take Me Already?

I read a book by Brian Tracy called the <u>Universal Laws of Success</u>. In it he wrote that when god wants to give you a gift, he wraps it up inside a problem. When you solve the problem, you realize the gift.

(Thank You Brian Tracy)

I wanted to die after my most recent dose of antibiotics sent my colitis into a flair to end all flairs. I was going to the bathroom every ½ hour all night long and the bowl was filled with bright red blood each time.

I asked the question "Why is god giving me all this pain and not taking my life?" My answer to the above question was, "Because he wants me to solve the problem, invent the cure and tell the world so others no longer have to suffer like I suffered."

Eventually, the antibiotic dose ran out and things seemed to get back to normal shortly after. Although normal for me was not normal for somebody else. Normal for me was 1-2 tablespoons of blood in each bowel movement and 5 or more movements a day. But at least I was not in severe pain all night long and I began getting several hours sleep at a clip per night.

I knew though that I was gonna cure it this time. I was gonna do research and make it my primary focus and turn over every leaf again and again until I found the gift God wanted me to find.

Chapter 9

How Can I Cure Myself By Christmas?

So, at this point I'm in I think my 11th year of having colitis and I asked the question, "How can I cure myself of Colitis and have fun in the process?"

And the magic happened, just like Tony Robbins said it would.

Answers started popping into my head. One of the first was that I had to figure out what it was that was actually causing this. I had to find the underlying cause. If I could figure that out, then I would have an actual enemy to attack. As it was, there was no known enemy except my immune system and attacking my defenses did not make sense, so it had to be something else causing this.

And then once I have an enemy to attack, then I can employ tactics I learned from reading a book called <u>A Champions Mind</u>, by tennis great, Pete Sampras.

In his book, he wrote that the way to beat your opponent is not to play your basic strengths, but rather, to play your *relative* strengths. That means: find what skills you have that are better than the same skills the opponent has and keep playing to those. So if you have a strong backhand and your opponent has a strong backhand, don't play your strong backhand to his strong backhand. If you have a weak forehand, but its better than his forehand, play your weak forehand to his weaker forehand.

This wisdom helped me come up with the cure for my Colitis.

(Thank you Pete Sampras)

SO WHAT'S THE CURE?

Well, first you need to know what the cause is. It's amazingly simple, so simple I overlooked it early on. Back then, there was talk about Candida and Leaky Gut Syndrome and imbalanced Flora and good bacteria vs bad bacteria in the intestine and it was all too unbelievable and overwhelming to me back then. Plus, I could find no one who ever said they were cured by fixing the imbalance. And since I thought antibiotics wiped out all bacteria, bugs and what not, that make up the flora, how could there be an imbalance of flora? It didn't make sense. Antibiotics I've had before, should allow me to start over and normal balance should ensue, thereafter – at least, that's what I thought then.

But 10 years later, it turns out that that simple imbalance in intestinal flora is the root of all my ails for the past 10 years. Antibiotics don't kill off all the flora, as I will eventually learn 10 years later.

So, I will explain the imbalance issue further in a minute, but knowing that it is an imbalance issue, raises another question. What caused the imbalance?

Well, some say imbalanced gut flora is a product of one or more of the following:

Poor Diet
Stress
Antibiotic Use
Injury
Infection

Of those, I believe Antibiotics is the primary instigator of the imbalance and let me explain why.

Firstly, there are case studies that show prolonged use of antibiotics leads to systemic yeast infection.

What is systemic Yeast infection and how do antibiotics cause that?

Well, antibiotics are great at killing bacteria which live normally in the intestines, however they are not so great at killing yeast that also naturally live in the intestines.

Why don't antibiotics kill yeast too? Because Yeast cells have an outer cellular structure that protects them from antibiotics, whereas bacteria do not have an outer protective shell.

Secondly, the last dose of antibiotics I took, sent me into a major flair. In the past, I never put the 2 together. I just thought it was because I was sick that I was flairing and antibiotics were supposed to be helping me. I just needed to kick the cold and colitis symptoms would ease up a bit, so I thought.

Thinking back, it was shortly after I took my first dose of antibiotics back in Arizona 10 years ago, that I first found blood in my stool.

However, I also think it takes more than just an instigator to get the imbalance happening. For instance, in Canada, it is a law that anyone administered antibiotics, must immediately receive a week long course of probiotics, namely BIO K, which is a mixture of live good bacteria and has proven to reduce the number of repeat visits by patients.

I think to get the imbalance really happening, it takes the instigator plus a lack of replenished bacteria, plus, a diet that Yeast thrive upon.

What happens is, normally, bacteria and yeast coexist in the intestines, at a ratio of about 80% bacteria, 20% Yeast. They compete for the resources that arrive in the intestines from the food we eat.

Bacteria normally keeps yeast in check, but a sudden lack of bacteria, allows Yeast to eat all it wants, and subsequently multiply very rapidly, taking over the intestines.

If you've ever seen dough rise during bread-making, you have an idea of how fast yeast can multiply, given the right environment. OR if you've ever left an orange on the counter for a week, all along it seems fine, then one day, its loaded with mold, aka fungus, aka yeast!

Bread is made by mixing live yeast with sugar and warm water in a bed of flour dough. The dough rises within minutes because the yeast start munching on the sugar and natural carbohydrates found in the dough – the yeast multiply like mad, releasing gas as they eat. The gas gets trapped in the flour, causing it to rise.

MIRACLE GROW FOR YEAST

So, take away the bacteria that keeps yeast in check in the intestines and add stuff that yeast love to eat (beer, vinegar, sugar, cheese) and what do you get? An imbalance in gut flora. So what's so bad about an imbalance of gut flora?

Well I'm sure you've heard of yeast infections? Women get them in their vagina often and are told to douche with probiotics to get rid of them. It causes foul smells and severe itching. And this is because the Yeast release gases and other compounds when they eat, that are dangerously different from those released by bacteria.

In addition, yeast can take root in the host cell walls, such as the inside of the vagina or intestines. When they do, they can then pull in substances that help them grow and the stuff they release is then released on the other side of the host cells, namely into the bloodstream of the victim. In other words, alcohol and other toxins the yeast produce are now pushed directly into the bloodstream and the body and liver become overloaded trying to combat these otherwise undesirable substances from the bloodstream.

This leaves little resources available to the liver to do its normal job of producing digestive enzymes to help break down the food we eat.

Subsequently, we are unable to utilize most of the food we eat and it instead becomes food for the yeast or exits the rectum unprocessed.

It becomes a vicious cycle, in that, less nutrients are absorbed by the body from food and more toxins enter our bloodstream every time we eat. This explains why I would do better by not eating. Unknowingly, I was starving the yeast and they could not multiply and the rate of toxins they dumped in my bloodstream would slow down.

INFLAMMATION IS GOOD

With this overload, of yeast in my intestines and toxins getting through my intestinal walls, my body tried to defend against the damage, the last way it knew how, via coating the interior walls of my intestines with a thick milky white mucous and heating up the intestinal walls, trying to kill off and block the offensive that was happening – basically: plug the windows and set the building on fire, should kill the bugs.

Unfortunately, the heat the body produces is not strong enough to kill yeast; they can survive at 120+ degrees or more, and the body can produce only so much mucous to block the holes, because it is too busy clearing out the toxins in the bloodstream and unfortunately it is not getting enough of a supply of nutrients.

It's like trying to fight a war, where you know you need 10,000 bullets to get the job done, but you only have 100. You do what you can. Unfortunately, this is a losing battle from the start. A valiant effort, but a losing one, none-the-less.

A side effect of the mucous is that it also blocks any nutrients from getting into the bloodstream.

A side effect of the heat the body is producing in the intestines is that the intestine walls can only take the heat for a short while before they begin to burn, and become ulcerated. The ulcers then bleed and wallah! -there's blood in my stool and in the toilet bowl.

IT JUST KEEPS GETTING BETTER

Now that blood is leaking out of the ulcers in my intestines, the body has to work even harder to do things it normally does, stealing resources from muscles, bones and other stores to repair intestinal walls and keep things working properly.

The intestines are normally the biggest user of glutamine, a substance which helps them regrow their cells on a regular basis. Just like we shed skin everyday which grows back, the intestines do the same. The body gets glutamine from its muscles, but after an injury, it can't get enough glutamine fast enough and so it is required via food sources.

CABBAGE FOR POPEYE?

Thus, they call glutamine a conditionally essential amino acid, You only need it from food when you have an injury. It's like Spinach for Popeye. It always gets him out of a jam and when he's in a jam is the only time he seems to eat it. (Oh Popeye, Oh. Holds on sweet peas, I'll's be rights there)) Studies show that glutamine supplementation helps burn victims heal more rapidly.

Green Cabbage is loaded with Glutamine, as well as having all the essential amino acids that the body can't produce on its own. Cabbage also tastes pretty bitter, but I've grown to love it.

There's also a study done in the 1950's that shows that fresh Cabbage Juice cured ulcers in 10 days.

Back to the death spiral... So now that blood is pouring out of me on a daily basis, my supply of iron begins to drop. And I seem to get along fine, until one day, my body runs out of iron and things start to shut down and you find yourself in the emergency room with a severe headache, chest pains, dizziness and no energy whatsoever. And your wife is pissed. And the doctors give you an infusion and tell you to take iron pills. And then you go home and start taking iron pills and eating lots of red meat because meat contains iron and the iron pills cause severe stomach pain and make you have diarrhea and now, no nutrition is getting in at all and you become dehydrated worse than before from all the diarrhea.

And then you throw in the towel and decide not to eat or drink anything, and a few days later you start to feel a little better. So, then you go and have a big meal and Bam! Back on the Porcelain Horse. Somehow you survive. But little by little your weight and will-power drop and it's just a matter of time before you are at the end of your rope.

ITS A WONDERFUL LIFE

"Help me Clarence. Help me get back.
I want to live again. I want to live again"
(George Bailey)

What a great day it was when I declared myself cured of Colitis. I told my wife and she said

"That would be so great if you had a cure for Christmas." And that's where the title for this book came about.

So it's no longer a wonderful life for the yeast that once overloaded my intestines. It's now a balanced life for them, living in harmony with the other bacteria I put back into my intestines. And its a wonderful life for me, finally.

So how did I discover this was a yeast infection? I read the book 8 Weeks to Optimum Health, by Dr Weil, who said to seek out others who self-healed themselves.

Shortly after that, I was researching complications from Ulcerative Colitis in the Natural Healing textbook and I saw that Oral Thrush was one complication. And it said it was caused by an overgrowth of Candida in the body, a yeast, and it can be relieved with anti-fungal medicine, ie. yeast killers.

Since I often had mouth and tongue sores during the past 10 years, bells went off in my head. Could it be that simple? Could an overgrowth of Yeast be causing my Colitis?

I searched google for the phrase "colitis yeast" and I came across one person who said they went on an anti-yeast diet and her colitis symptoms had disappeared in 10 days.

(Thank you Google)

But it was all so very vague. No contact information was provided about the person.

I searched for the difference between yeast and bacteria, cause I thought they were one in the same. Turns out, they were far from the same. I learned that antibiotics kill bacteria, not yeast and when that happens, yeast can grow like wildfire.

I looked up thrush cures on google and found someone who had a 3Day Thrush Cure. I bought her ebook and learned what she used for anti-fungals and bacteria replenishment, as well as some of her diet recipes. Her methods cured her and her baby of Oral Thrush, rapidly. Could it work for Ulcerative Colitis too?

(Thank you Rebecca Haworth)

"HOLY CRAP BATMAN – You really stepped in it this time."

(3rd grade humor flashback)

I remembered a stool test I had done when this first hit me 10 years ago. Dr Stengler, had me collect a sample of my poop (that was fun!) and put it in a vile and mail out to a place called Great Smokies Lab, now called Genova Diagnostics.

They analyzed it and gave me a report on the balance of gut flora that they found in it. I had long lost this report, but remembered there was something about Saccharomyces in it.

And as I recently began researching yeast, I kept running into the word Saccharomyces. I remember not fully understanding 10 years ago, what it was and I remember ordering something that was supposed to help replenish it - something called Sacchoromyces Boulardi. I took a bottle of the pills over the course of a few weeks back then. Turns out, that was a huge mistake. I had read the report wrong.

I recently retrieved the old report from Dr Stengler's office and took another look. Now it all made total sense. I spoke Yeast Science now, thanks to all the research I recently did and now I could understand the report better.

"I ALWAYS GET IT RIGHT IN THE END" -pun intended
(Myley Cirus)

My mistake was that the report said it found a problem with the balance of Sacchoromyces Cerevisiae and it could be retrieved with Sacchormyces Boulardi.. I thought it meant I was supposed to supplement my diet with Boulardi to fix the balance. But what it really meant was Boulardi could be mistaken as Cerevisiae, because of the similarities in how they detect Cerevisiae and Boulardi.

I was not supposed to add Boulardi. The report said I had too much Cerevisiae and not enough Bifidum. To be clear, Cerevisiae and Boulardi are yeast cells, Bifidum is bacteria cells.

It said my level of Cerevisiae was pathogenic, meaning I was in trouble because of an overgrowth of yeast and a shortage of bacteria and the yeast is doing damage. And there I was, adding more yeast to my already yeast-overloaded intestine. That was a fun time, let me tell ya. If the toilet bowl could talk...

Like I said, at the time, I though all bugs fell into the same category and they were all called bacteria, also referred to as gut flora, but that so is not the case. There's a big difference between yeast cells and bacteria cells that live in the intestines.

I am not sure back them if anyone knew how to treat yeast overgrowth and I remember the Natural Doctor having me eat crockpot meals. But I remember I was putting lots of carrots, onions, and potatoes in the recipes and that is certainly food for the yeast. Those foods are loaded with carbohydrates, which yeasts thrive on. And that explains why my crockpot cooking experiments did not work for me.

Anyhow, after rereading the Great Smokies report, it was clear and made total sense that my body was trying to defend itself against a yeast overgrowth, aka infection.

(Thank you Great Smokies & Dr. Stengler)

Now, armed with all this knowledge, I started to experiment with an Anti-Yeast diet and Bio K and noticed marked improvement within days.

But some days I was having severe problems. I knew I was close, but something still was not perfect yet.

I was alternating days with lots of Raw Garlic and Grapefruit Seed Extract I was told they both kill yeast. But it turns out after looking up garlic on NutritionDATA.com, garlic is mainly carbohydrates and thus more food for yeast. The oil could be good, but eating the whole cloves caused problems for me.

(Thank You NutritionData.com)

So I cut out the Garlic and symptoms started becoming stable. I also cut out the Grapefruit Seed Extract because of stuff I read about it on the internet.

MAGIC BULLETS

I did more research on the life of yeast. I found a very helpful Wikipedia article

(Thank you Wikipedia & Contributors).

It turns out yeast slow down or die when confronted with salt or butter.

It struck a chord, because a couple of days earlier I had a meal where I mixed some coconut oil I bought for a recipe in the 3 day thrush book, in with some macadamia nuts and hazelnuts. And I sensed that something was magical about that coconut oil. Coconut Oil is fatty just like butter, so maybe the 2 have a similar affect on Yeast. I was afraid of butter.

I did some research on coconut oil and found that it is often used as a reliable disinfectant. It has an oil that is a short chain fatty acid, small enough to slip through and penetrate the tough outer shells of yeast cells. And since it's just the oil of the coconut, the sugar part has been removed, and the oil won't feed yeast.

Salt also struck a chord, because a recent bout with strep throat had me search for a method to ease the severe pain in my throat. I came across a YouTube video of someone showing that all you had to do was just shake some salt onto the back of your throat and he explained that salt draws out the water from the bad bug cells and then the rest of the cell implodes by its own enzymes and dies, killing the bugs and thus easing the pain. I had tried it and it worked on my throat.

(Thank You YouTube Guy)

So then I decided, why not mix salt with coconut oil and hit the yeast with a two-punch combination?

I loaded up on the stuff, 2-4 tablespoons a day. I would mix a tablespoon in with a bowl of macadamia nuts, hazelnuts and sesame seeds and lots of sea salt. It tastes yummy . I picked nuts that were high in fat and low in carbohydrates, so not to feed the yeast and do more to beat them up.

STING LIKE A BEE

"Come on Gorilla. This is a Thrilla"
Muhammad Ali

(I wonder if Gorillas eat honey and get stung by bees and it keeps them healthy? I digress. .Anyhow...)

So, after doing the rope-a-dope for 10 years, I finally figured out how to fight colitis. I had my opponent up against the ropes in the corner. I finally knew its name. Yeast. I found the Cause of Colitis I was looking for and now I knew its strengths and weaknesses.

However, those yeast are tough like Joe Frazier. They don't give up easily. I had to figure a way to knock 'em out - just like Muhammad Ali knew how to float like a butterfly and sting like a bee and beat Frazier in some of the toughest fights in history.

Now I had my shot at the title. And here's where I put it all together.

"But Apollo, you taught me everything you know."
Rocky

"Not everything. Not everything."
Apollo Creed

I found one more final Magic Bullet. Dr Weil's book mentioned a case about a person who claims to have been cured of colitis after having been stung by a bee in the knee.

As I was researching yeast, and enzymes used to help make yeast grow, I came across the word peptide, and found out peptides were cleaved Amino Acids, or Proteins, reassembled in many different ways. And they can act like friends or foes to yeast according to their particular design.

Turns out, many medicines are made from production of certain peptide combinations. So in essence, I just need to find or produce the right combination of amino acid parts.

I thought I could eat enzymes with protein and that would possibly create the right peptides I needed to beat up the yeast some more. But that was a long shot and I'm no chemist.

Luckily however, I found a link in my research about a peptide compound found naturally in bee venom. Another bell went off. I dug some more. It said a compound similar to Melittin, the primary compound found in bee venom was significantly effective in preventing yeast growth, in preventing yeast cells from taking root in intestine walls and in soaking up yeast cells and destroying them.

So, all I needed to do was get stung by a bee.

A little more research into bee stings and I found that when the venom hits the bloodstream, it causes the brain to produce lots of Cortisol. Cortisol is a natural and super powerful steroid. I thought, "I could use that!"

I learned people were getting regular bee stings in Los Angeles and it was helping their Multiple Sclerosis. Body parts that did not move properly, suddenly came to life after getting stung by a bee. I saw a video about it on YouTube and I became a believer.

Unfortunately LA is 2 hours from me and the doctor doing it only does it Monday, Tuesday and Wednesday mornings and it costs a lot.

I did some more digging as to where I could get this done. It turns out that in New Zealand, they patented a way to get the bee venom out of bees without killing them. Normally, when a bee stings a human, the bee dies because the stinger and sack separate from the bee and stay stuck to the human.

However, the New Zealand process uses a method where bees are in a box on a sheet of glass and the glass has electrodes on it. A small shock is sent through and the bees get alarmed and sting the glass. Their stinger does not separate. Then the bees are shaken off the glass and what remains is bee venom. The bees live on and the venom is left to dry on the glass. The dried venom is then scraped off and put it into tablets.

(Thank you New Zealand)

And guess what? I could order the tablets in the mail! And I did. They are called ApiVenz and each tablet contains ½ a bee stings worth of venom.

So now, I had a known enemy, I knew its strengths and weaknesses and I was heavily armed. Using Sampras' mindset, I put together a relative strengths and weaknesses game plan. I realized that the human body can thrive on Fat, but Yeast can't. I can handle salt fine, Yeast can't.   Yeast love carbohydrates, vinegar, alcohol, & moldy foods. I can get along fine without those.

If I'm not allergic to bee stings, I have another weapon against the yeast.

Fortunately, I'm not allergic to bee stings.   I was once stung by a bee about 20 years ago and, though it hurt like a son of a gun and I had the typical swelling and a scar to prove it, I did not go into shock. Thus I was armed to the hill. It was fight time.

"Ding, Ding."

Apollo Creed

So, I did what I always did. I went full force. I ran out to my local health food store, Jimbo's and got most of the stuff I needed from them. Then I went online and ordered some other stuff I needed and then I got busy treating myself.

(Thank you Jimbo's)

I am putting all the stuff I did, and did not do in the appendix, along with resource links & recipes.   I also created a site for all the links too. It's http://10DayColitisCure.com

Obviously I make money on the sale of this book, and some of the products I link to on my site and I hope you are OK with that. I wanted to be a writer and now I am, and I think it's OK, healthy, and necessary to profit from what you love to do and if you can help others. I wish everyone could do the same.

THE OBLIGATORY DISCLAIMER

And please don't sue me, because obviously I am not a doctor. This book is simply an account of how I think I cured myself, not necessarily a cure for anyone else and it is not medical advice. Always seek advice from your doctor before undertaking any new program. (There Denny Crane, are we in the clear?)

WIN ROCKY WIN

"Yo Adrian, I did it. I did it!"

Rocky

And the winner is...

Cue the music. ("Gonna fly Now!")

I kicked yeasts ass. 10 days later, my poop was looking really good. I was sleeping through the night. No pain. No stomach gurgling. No rushing to the bathroom. One, maybe 2 bowel movements a day. Some days no bowel movements at all. It was incredible.

"SCRATCH THAT ITCH"

Devo

On the 2nd day of this new regime, I was getting into bed for the night and I felt itchy all over. I scratched but couldn't find where it was. I scratched and scratched and finally went to sleep. The next morning I looked up 'body itch' on the internet and found cases where they said it was a sign of massive yeast die-off. I was psyched!

The itching went away the next day and never came back.

Around the 4th day, I had a strange color green poop come out and I researched that and it said that green poop is a sign of clearing out the last of an infection. What happens is a lot of bile is released by the liver to help clean out the dead bugs leftover from a serious infection. Bile is green. It means my liver is functioning well, now that it's no longer overloaded fighting the alcohol and other toxins the yeast were dumping into my bloodstream rivers.

When I read that, that's when I raised my arms in victory, jumped up and down and declared myself cured.

The next morning I woke up in bed and cried like a baby. 10 years of emotional roller coasters, cured in less than 10 days. I was angry, happy, relieved, sad, 10 different emotions flooding me all at once. I couldn't control myself and I let it all out and vowed to tell the world so it never happens to any one else ever again. No one should have to go through what I went through. 10 years of my life were lost.

A few days later, I had major diarrhea, but no blood , no pain. It smelled like sauerkraut. I looked it up on the internet and found that initiating a course of probiotics can cause diarrhea at first, but then it goes away as your body adapts. And sure enough, no more diarrhea after that. I still have sauerkraut smelling movements but I can live with that. I was healed and happier than a pig in poop.

I sat down a few weeks later and began writing this book.

When this book is in your hands, which it is if you are reading this now, then my mission is complete. I received a great gift and am passing it on. Please do the same for anyone you know who may be suffering.

(Thank YOU Reader!)

Chapter 10

Why Didn't I Learn This 10 Years Ago?

A few years back, I had read the book, <u>Mans Search For Meaning</u>, by Victor Frankl and in it the author/psychologist talks about how only a few people survived the Holocaust, him being one of them.

He claims that it was because he convinced himself that his purpose in life was to survive and tell the story of the atrocities that occurred, so to prevent it from ever happening again and to tell others about how to determine their own meaning of life, so they can thrive.

This way of thinking helped me do what I did. I kept visioning writing this book – it meant I had to first find a cure and eventually, I did it!

(Thank you Dr Frankl)

So why didn't I learn this cure 10 years ago? Because 10 years ago, I would not have written this book and I wanted to be a writer but never took the chance and probably never would have if not for the desire to save people from this affliction. It was Gods gift that I was stricken with this sickness. He put me here for a reason and discovering this cure is one of them. Also, it let me be the writer I wanted to be. That is my belief anyhow and that is what got me through in the end. (no pun intended)

(Thanks Again God)

At the time of this writing, I've actually written a screenplay, which I submitted to the Writers Network Fiction Competition and so far, I made it to the quarter finals. My script is called Century Ever After. I'm crossing my fingers that it will make it to the finals and then I may get phone calls from agents wanting me to write more screenplays. Wish me luck.

As for now, thanks for reading and if you haven't already, I wish you all find your meaning of life and thrive. I hope this book was helpful.

I can be reached at mwkanter@yahoo.com or mwkanter@gmail.com

I'd love to hear from you and how you are doing. (So long as you're not a sicko stalker of some kind ;)

Be Well & Don't Quit!
Mark

Appendix A

Resources, Recipes & Regimen

RESOURCES

I created a site that has links to this book and most of the stuff I bought . It's http://10DayColitisCure.com

OK, the stuff I bought to replenish the bacteria in my intestines was from 2 places. One I purchased at Jimbos. It is called Bio-K+ Plus. They have several varieties, I chose the dairy free one as I just never have luck with dairy. It's the purple bottles. They keep them in the fridge at the store. It's expensive.

The dairy free one has nutritional yeast in addition to the lactobacillus strains of bacteria. I was a little concerned at first and still am and therefore prefer to get my bacteria naturally by making my own homemade sauerkraut.

Nutrional Yeast is dead Sacchoromyces Cerivisiae. It is loaded with b vitamins and is very tasty, but it's what I was trying to get rid of. I think it is supposed to help the lactobacillus grow. BioK+ makes other dairy varieties that don't have that nutritional yeast added.

Sauerkraut is just raw cabbage and salt. I bought organic raw cabbage and a homemade sauerkraut maker. What happens is you chop up 5 heads of cabbage add 3 tablespoons of sea salt, mash it into the glass jar, put the special lid on, put it in 60-70 degree weather for 6 days and presto! - you now have a very inexpensive source of healthy bacteria to consume every day.

Plus its loaded with glutamine, enzymes, and all your essential amino acid proteins to help repair intestinal damage.

I was told if I buy sauerkraut from the store, it may have been pasteurized/heated and the bacteria would be dead and the enzymes and other good stuff could be rendered useless.

So I bought the maker, made my own and its delicious. Makes for good farts too! Impress all your friends!!

Jimbos:
http://www.jimbos.com/

BioK:

http://www.biokplus.com/en/

Sauerkraut Maker:
http://store.therawdiet.com/pisaandkimch.html

Sauerkraut Making Instructions:
http://www.therawdiet.com/pdf/KrautInstructions.pdf

I bought the bee sting venom tablets via internet mail order here:

ApiVenz:
http://beevenomtherapy.biz/ApiVenz_Tablets.ht m

I bought Organic Raw Virgin Coconut Oil at Henry's Farmers Market

Coconut Oil at Henry's:
http://www.henrysmarkets.com

or here's 2 other resources
http://www.vitacost.com/Nutiva-Organic-Extra-Virgin-Coconut-Oil-15-oz?csrc=GPF-692752200014

http://www.vitaminshoppe.com/store/en/browse/sku_detail.jsp?id=GU-7001&sourceType=cs&source=FG&cm_mmc=Shopping%20Engines-_-googleproduct-_-Coconut%20Oil%20Extra%20Virgin%20/%20Organic%20-

%2016%20Ounces%20Solid-_-GU-
7001&ci_src=14110944&ci_sku=GU-7001

I bought Raw Organic Macadamias, Hazelntus and
Unhulled Sesame Seeds at Jimbos from their bins. I
buy enough for a week at a time, so they are fresh as I
can get them.

High Fat/Low Carb Nuts and Seeds:
http://www.jimbos.com/

here's 2 more resources:
http://www.healthyfoodmall.com/natural-
organic-nuts

http://www.nutsonline.com/cookingbaking/seed
s/sesame/natural.html?
gclid=CKGMx4HBjZ4CFShGagodIyEHtg

I bought REAL Sea Salt at Jimbo's

here's another source
http://www.myhealthpro.com/shop/detail.cfm?
sku=D0930&rfr=FRG&zmam=1000941&zmas=24&
zmac=114&zmap=D0930

I bought Pau D' Arco Tea from Jimbos

Here's some other resources:

http://www.google.com/products?
q=Pau+D'+Arco+Tea&rls=com.microsoft:en-
us:IE-SearchBox&oe=UTF-
8&sourceid=ie7&rlz=1I7GWYE_en&um=1&ie=U
TF-8&ei=8ToAS_bcII7ysQOBv-
2dCg&sa=X&oi=product_result_group&ct=title&
resnum=4&ved=0CC0QrQQwAw

I bought frozen shrimp peeled without tail at
Costco. The only other ingredient added is salt.
And Salt helps kill yeast. I don't think they sell it
online. It's the orange bag. They are 50-70
shrimp per pound. Their size seems to taste
better to me than the larger or smaller sized
shrimp.

Costco:
http://www.costco.com/

RECIPES

DEANNA'S MAGIC MEAL

(1 bowl in morning, 1 bowl in evening)
Ingredients:
Handful of organic raw Macadamias,
Handful of organic Hazelnuts/Filberts
Handful of Organic Raw Unhulled Sesame Seeds
1-2 Tblsp Organic Virgin Coconut Oil
Salt to taste – go heavy

Directions:
Mix all with a spoon in a small bowl and eat.
(sprinkle more salt as you go if loses salt taste)

This is the main meal I eat. I love it and my body loves it and the yeast hate it. It takes the same amount of time to make as a bowl of cereal. I have it at breakfast and as a snack at night when watching TV. Better than pocorn.

I named it after my daughter, because I get to eat breakfast with her now and snack during TV time with her while she either has a bowl of cereal or popcorn. She says it smells much better than that other stuff I used to eat. (blah!) Sometimes I poor Coconut milk into it and I swear its the best tasting cereal ever.

MARK'S COCONUT SHRIMP

Ingredients:

20 Frozen Costco Shrimp
1 Tablespoon Coconut Oil
Salt to Taste

Instructions:
Put Shrimp in a bowl, microwave for almost 2 minutes. Remove from microwave, mix in Coconut oil and Sea Salt with a spoon and eat.

This takes the same amount of time as making cereal or oatmeal and it is my favorite meal. Seriously, it is delicious. Sometimes I have it without the Coconut Oil. I am a huge fan of Shrimp, so I named this one after myself.

NANA'S WALNUT SALAD

Ingredients:

1 plate of Spinach
2 roma tomatoes in chunky slices
Handful of Walnuts
Salt to Taste

Instructions:
Layer a plate with raw spinach. Slice up 2 organic Roma tomatoes to desired thickness. I like mine chunky. Sprinkle lots of walnuts over the top. Sprinkle Lots of Sea Salt over the top and eat.

This is surprisingly simple and delicious and loaded with good stuff. My mom used to eat tomatoes with salt like she was eating an easter egg. I had forgotten how good tomatoes with just salt can taste. The added walnuts with salt really takes this over the top.

(Thanks Mom)

SPIKES STEAK

Ingredients:

Filet Mignon
Braggs Liquid Aminos
Salt to taste

Instructions:
Fry up or bake the Filet Mignon with salt and
Braggs Liquid Aminos and eat with Rebeccas
SauerKraut. Pour some more salt and Braggs
over the meal as you eat to keep it extra salty.
Yeast hate that.

I named this recipe after Spike the Dinosaur,
one of my daughter's favorite toys that Nana
bought her for Christmas last year. We have a
blast with that mighty, miniature, meat eater.

I eat it with Rebeccas Sauerkraut because the
bacteria help break down the meat and meat is
usually tough to eat. I try not to eat the fat parts
of the meat because animal fats usually contain
lots of toxins, its the place the mammal bodies
stores toxins. Plus I don't really like the taste of
the fat on the steak.

REBECCAS SAUERKRAUT

Ingredients:
5 heads of organic cabbage
3 tablespoons sea salt

Instructions:
Shred the cabbage, mix with salt in a gigantic bowl . Pack it down into the glass jar. Seal as instructed in the homemade sauerkraut maker instructions.   Let sit outside in 60-70 degree weather for 6 days until the bubbles stop. Refrigerate and eat.

I named this one after Rebecca Haworth who put out the 3 day thrush cure which had recommended this to cure yeast infections. It's delicious and I think probably one of the healthiest foods on the planet. It's how our ancestors used to survive through the winter when there was no refrigeration or vegetation. The stuff lasts for months. She has lots more yummy anti-yeast recipes in her e-book.

3 Day Thrush Cure – you can get it here: http://0b4bd13iromi9oc44eromgzcx1.hop.clickbank.net/?tid=COLITIS

or via link from my site
http://10DayColitisCure.com

You probably noticed a theme with all the recipes I use. They take like 2 minutes to make max. I like convenience and found healthy meals that work for my style.

Coconut Oil I use like butter in place of it, I just need to add a bunch of salt to it and it tastes 10xs better and it is 10xs better health-wise in my opinion.

KARINS COLADA

Ingredients:

8 Ice cubes
¼ cup coconut milk
1/2 tsp salt
½ tsp Cream of Tartar

Instructions:

Blend all ingredients in a powerful blender and
enjoy it like it was a Pina Colada

I read that Cream of Tartar Kills yeast and its
sweet tasting. It's whats left after grapes ferment
into wine, so I guess the bacteria took all the
edible carbs and left behind unedible ones?

REGIMEN

THE SAMPRAS GAME PLAN

Play Your Bodies Relative Strengths Against the Yeast

1. <u>Starve the Yeast so they stop multiplying</u>

This is done with a 2 week diet that avoids yeasts favorite foods

So, Eat Like the Atkins Diet (High Fat/Protein, Low Carbs) but also:

No Vinegar foods (which is most condiments, like mustard, ketchup etc),

No Moldy Foods (ie. No leftovers, no cheese, no Eggs, no pistachios, no cashews, no potatoes, no mushrooms, no rice),

No Alcohol,

No Milk,

No sugar,

No Flour,

No Corn,

No Fruit,

No Fruit Juice,

No Soy,

No fermented foods (pickles,yogurt,sour cream),
No Flax,
no cans,
no beans

2.Kill the Yeast

This is done with natural Anti-fungals

1.Sea Salt. (load up on this)

2.Organic Virgin Coconut Oil (2-4 tablespoons a day) or eat 2 bowls of the Magic Meal recipe

3.Pau D' Arco Tea (3 cups a day)

3.Soak up and flush out the Dying Yeast

1.Sesame Seeds

2.Bee Venom (2 tablets day, dissolve under tongue - don't swallow, no food/water for ½ hour after)

4.Replenish Good Bacteria

1.Bio K (Dairy Free) 1 dose a day or

2.Homemade Sauerkraut (1 bowl a day) (better than Bio k)

5.Heal Intestinal Damage & Block Future Damage

1.Bee Venom

2.Cabbage Juice (blend ½ cabbage in blender a day and drink immediately)

3.Homemade Sauerkraut

In general, only eat twice a day to give more time for intestines to rest/heal between meals

Safe to Eat during these 2 weeks is:

All lean fresh meats (Beef, Pork, Chicken, Fish, Shrimp, Crab) Hormone free is best

All organic fresh, non-starchy, non-moldy herbs and vegies (Lettuce, Tomatoes,Red Peppers, Dill, Basil, cucumbers, eggplant, cabbage, romaine, spinach, asparagus, green beans, edame)

All organic raw non-moldy, low-carb nuts and seeds (macadamias, hazelnuts,walnuts, brazil nuts)

Sea Salt (lots)

Braggs Liquid Aminos

I avoid all spices except salt. Most spices are mainly carbohydrates, aka yeast food. Fresh Dill and Fresh Basil are good though. I eat them raw.

A KICK IN THE BUTT

I found that the last thing to disappear was the blood. I kept having a little bit at the end of my movements and then around the 2nd week I started giving myself a 2 Tablet Bee Venom suppository before I went to sleep at night. I did that for a few days and no longer. And the blood finally went away.

Gradually I reduced my Asacol medication and within a month I was down to 3 pills every other day. When I started I was taking 12 pills a day. By next month I will probably be totally off the medication.

I tried reintroducing carbohydrates, but when I did, I started noticing my stools getting worse so I backed off, just to be safe. I imagine it may take a long time before I can load up on carbohydrates again. And I will take it slow, if at all, because frankly, I truly don't feel I need them, nor do I really miss them.

The benefit of eating lots of nuts and seeds instead of a carb loaded diet has been that the nuts fill me up fast. I feel satisfied for a long time and therefore, I need to spend less time eating to thrive. I eat twice a day now. As a result, I have more time to do the other things I want to do in life, like writing, investing, and playing games with family and friends. It's a great trade.

Appendix B

Eating Out

Some of the hardest parts about sticking to a diet of any kind is handling situations where you go out to eat with others.

Nowadays it's pretty easy and acceptable to tell people you are following the Atkins diet. Many restaurants have a section to help people on that diet. So when I am out, I look for the meals that are recommended on the menu for those who are counting carbohydrates. And then I ask the waiter to substitute anything that I know is a yeast favorite. If they can't, I simply just don't eat the problem items.

Examples of what I order at places I go out:

Panda Express:
I get the steamed vegies instead of the rice and noodles and ask them to aim for the broccoli. I get tai cashew chicken, green bean chicken or mandarin chicken. I avoid the breaded stuff.

Chevy's Mexican Grill
I get the Chicken, Shrimp or Steak Fajita with sauteed vegies. I avoid the chips, tortillas,

beans, sour cream , salsa and rice. I sometimes eat the Guacomole.

Lil Pepper Deli
I get a grilled chicken salad, no sauces. I ask for dressing on the side and just avoid it. I also avoid the croutons and carrots.

Outback Steakhouse
I get a steak of any sort, or crablegs. Steamed vegies. I avoid the potatoes, bread, and any breaded stuff. I get a salad with sauce on the side and ask for no cheese.

Chilis
I get the Chicken Wings and avoid the dipping sauces. I get a Grilled Chicken Salad.

Fillipis Italian Pizza Grotto
I get a salad with dressing on the side. I avoid the croutons, carrots, onions and the dressing. I have the most trouble at italian restaurants as almost everything comes loaded with carbs. I often avoid Italian restaurants as a result.

Denny's
I get a grilled chicken entree with sliced tomatoes, coleslaw and a skewer of grilled shrimp. I smother it all in salt.

A good way I like to think of how I need to eat is, that I pretend to myself that I am simply allergic to carbs,dairy and vinegar. The rest is then easy.

Appendix C

My Daily Routine

During the first 10 days, here's what I did, did not do and the effects I saw along the way. I announced myself cured in the 3rd day and am little by little going to add back other stuff to my diet. But quite frankly, I don't miss anything from my old diet. I'm not craving anything and as a result, I have continued to stay on this diet as I truly enjoy it and feel quite strongly that it is the healthiest diet ever. I believe it will serve me well, and make me live well into my 100's.

So day 1 I went out and bought BioK+ dairy free, 5 heads of cabbage, macadamia nuts, hazelnuts, unhulled sesame seeds and Coconut Oil.

The BioK instructions said to start off with ¼ bottle of BioK, but the 3 day thrush book said to load up on probiotics at first, so I chose the advice of the latter. I chugged a bottle in the morning and a bottle at night.

I took 2 Bee Venom tablets and placed them under my tongue and let them dissolve there. I took them on my way out the door to work everday, so I wouldn't drink or eat anything for a half hour after. This is supposedly how it gets into the bloodstream without getting destroyed by the stomach acid and enzymes. I noticed a slight headache for a few minutes after taking them. It really wasn't that bad though. I imagine it was the Cortisol my brain was naturally producing and rushing it to help my intestines. So a little headache to me was worth it.

I made Rebeccas homemade cabbage and put it outside and let it ferment for 6 days, until I noticed it stopped bubbling. That's when I switched from drinking the BioK+ to eating the Sauerkraut.

I made a bowl of Deanna's Magic Meal for breakfast and dinner every day and if I was still hungry I would make a bowl of Mark's Coconut Shrimp and eat that too. I would also eat some sauerkraut as a snack or side with my meals. I would have Nana's Walnut Salad as a first course at dinner.

By the 2nd day, my poop changed color dramatically and blood seemed just about gone. I was astonished. Never had the blood disappeared that fast before. I had body itching that night.

I began having chopped raw garlic . But I started having gas pains and things began to get worse. So, I dropped the garlic and things got better quickly.

I began drinking the Pau D' Arco tea as directed, 3 cups a day while at my work. I really enjoy that too! It's the only thing I drink besides filtered water.

Stayed with this diet for the next 5 days. I was cured by the 3rd day in my mind. And I was no longer having headaches when I took the Bee Venom tablets.

On the 6th day, my Sauerkraut was done fermenting, so I started having it in place of the BioK+

I had major diarrhea for a few days and then things settled down and my poop starting looking really healthy.

I am a big ice chewing fan by the way, so a treat for myself is simply a cup of ice. I tried to get thin ice so it doesn't damage my teeth so much.

But it sure is a pleasure to me and mixes things up a bit.   I have quite a few cups every day.

I have a shower filter that filters out the chlorine from my water. I read that the skin absorbs the toxins from the chlorine water and so I never wanted to tax my liver more than necessary. Don't know if that makes a difference or not, but it feels good mentally at least. And I feel comfortable drinking the water in the shower if I'm thirsty during my shower. I picked the filter up at Jimbos, it was quite simple to screw on by hand. I change it every 6 months or so.

Appendix D

Future Research, Ideas & Other Acknowledgements

At the time of this writing, studies are being done at university hospitals, such as Georgetown University on the effects of Bee Venom on certain diseases. I hope that type of research continues.

It is pretty easy to find out the carbohydrate portion in foods in order to help prevent yeast growth. I used a site called NutritionData.com for many answers that helped guide my food choices.

http://NutritionData.com

I mainly look at 3 things on each food item. I check the grams of protein, grams of fat and grams of carbohydrates., if that ratio is more than 1/3rd carbohydrates, I try to avoid it. If the carbohydrate portion is less than 1/3 I will eat it. That is, unless I know for sure yeast thrive on it. For example. I avoid eggs and potatoes as I learned that they are often used quite successfully to grow yeast cultures in laboratories.

In Canada, they require you to take a course of probiotics for a week after you have a course of antibiotics. I think it should be taken a step further. I think while someone is taking antibiotics, they should be required to take 2-4 tablespoons of Coconut Oil a day, so to also kill off the yeast - not that they ever have a chance of getting the upper hand in the intestine. I know that I will eat Coconut Oil if ever I need another dose of antibiotics to get rid of a cold.

When I announced that I cured myself of Colitis, one of my best friends asked if I could now find the cure for that other C word, Cancer. My two best friends fathers, both died at an early age to that terrible disease, and so did several of my grandparents. I hope that the research being done on Cancer, looks into the possible effects of Bee Venom, Coconut Oil and Yeast on either curing or causing that horrible disease. Could there be a relation between the 2 diseases causes or cures? I wonder. And as Tony Robbins would say... I hope the researchers out there ask the right question of themselves and that is: "How Can I Find a Cure for Cancer by Christmas *AND* have fun in the process?"

OTHER ACKNOWLEDGEMENTS

My good friend, Mark Livolsi is designing a cover for the 2nd release of this book. He didn't care for the pink explosion, but my daughter loved it and it was easy to make using Cover Creator at CreateSpace.

> (Thank you Markay Markay & CreateSpace)

My brother Wayne's words of encouragement, helped me get up off the canvas when I didn't have it in me anymore.

> (Thank You Bro)

My daughter Deanna's future dreams, kept me alive. I believe she will become the Tennis Rockstar she wants to be, or whatever she may change her mind to want to be and I want to give her all the support I can to reach her dreams.

> (Thank you Sweetie)

My wife Karin, put up with the roller coaster more than I think anyone else ever could. She deserves an award and I wish there were a way I could give her back the 10 years that she lost helping me battle this terrible disease.

(Thank you Honey)

My good friend, Bob Farulla, kept sending me
songs from our glory days in High School. It
gave me many needed boosts along the way. I
have them saved on my VoiceMail and listen to
them often.

(Thank You Buddy)

After 10 long years of battling Ulcerative Colitis,
a debilitating and demoralizing
disease that affects the intestines, causing
embarrassing urgent bowel movements,
bloody stools and steady decrease in nutrient
absorption, slowly destroying the
will, confidence and spirit of an otherwise
healthy-on-the-outside-appearing person,
Mark Kanter finally figured out the science
behind what caused his supposed, cause-
unknown, incurable illness and invented a cure
for himself he would like to share
with the 1 in 10,000 people afflicted with this
silent destroyer.

Mark Kanter lives in San Diego and is an expert
in Ulcerative Colitis, having had
the illness for more than 10 years and trying
everything under the sun to cure it.
He's tried crazy diets, enemas, mind-control,
acupuncture, homeopathy, steroids,
enzymes, NSAIDs, you name it. You won't
believe the lengths he's gone to to try and
beat this thing. Well, after 10 years of
experimenting on himself, he's proud to
finally announce the cure that lasts. Mark would
like to say to anyone who has or
has a friend with Colitis. IT CAN BE BEAT!